# MAMA SAID THERE'D BE DAYS LIKE THIS

## A Twelve Step Guide To Surviving A Mastectomy

Karen Klein

Introduction by
Peter Sugerman, M.D.

**Variegate Press**

Mama Said There'd Be Days Like This
A Twelve Step Guide To Surviving A Mastectomy

Copyright © 2004 by Karen Klein

Variegate Press
Farmington, CT

Library of Congress Control Number 2004102446
ISBN: 0-9749748-0-3

All rights reserved. No part of this publication may be reproduced without the prior permission of the author.

Printed in the United States of America

## CONTENTS

Introduction ............................................. 5
Author's Note ......................................... 11
Acknowledgements ................................. 13

Step 1   Choose Life ............................... 15
Step 2   Houston, We Have a Problem ..... 21
Step 3   The Eye of the Tiger .................. 27
Step 4   Pikes Peak or Bust ..................... 31
Step 5   'A' is for Adapting ..................... 35
Step 6   The Wise Warrior Woman .......... 39
Step 7   The Polyanna Principle ............. 43
Step 8   Mirror, Mirror ........................... 47
Step 9   Plan B ....................................... 53
Step 10  Nipples Optional ...................... 59
Step 11  Save the Last Dance ................. 65
Step 12  The Big Picture ........................ 71

Afterword ................................................ 79

## INTRODUCTION

If essays were rated like movies, *Mama Said There'd Be Days Like This,* would be rated "for mature audiences only." This unique discourse on how to cope with a mastectomy is a no-nonsense, penetrating, true account of one woman's experience of overcoming the emotional suffering of breast cancer surgery, presented in cognitive and behavioral chapters that are easy to understand. There are no wasted words, no attempts to disguise difficult feelings and issues, no pejorative phrasing. Such directness is not often found in self-help literature. Many may shy away from a direct approach because it creates discomfort, but for those who are brave, the end effect is that of instilling hope. It is hope founded on the promise that one's own efforts will be rewarded and that one can feel whole again.

*Mama Said There'd Be Days Like This* is a unique workbook. It encompasses a range of confusing, intense, or painful feelings and thoughts with which the mastectomy patient may have to deal. The intent of the author is to allow others to learn from what she discovered during her private struggle to cope with breast cancer. Those who are seriously grappling with their own issues concerning breast cancer or another cancer may be personally touched. Perhaps only one paragraph or phrase will connect, perhaps many, since each of us struggles in a unique way. Others may simply be inspired by the strength of character portrayed or be inspired to reach more deeply into their own personal struggles. Still others may only strive to understand the types of issues and emotions with which the mastectomy survivor is dealing.

It is an honor to submit an introduction for this breast cancer survival manual. Knowing the author as a friend for over twenty years, I find this discourse to represent an accurate reflection of her character. She worked hard to become whole again, not just for herself but for her children, her family, and for anyone who may care about such matters. She did not stop until she saw this undertaking through to its completion.

My contribution to this work is more academic. I will attempt to describe how the issues of coping with breast cancer appear from the perspective of a psychiatrist. I have practiced in the Hartford, Connecticut area for over fifteen years. What I find most notable about the psychology of breast cancer and mastectomies is the unique complexity of emotions that mastectomy surgery stirs up in an individual. This uniqueness is not intuitively obvious. On the surface, breast cancer is only one of several serious cancers that may shorten a life span; and since a mastectomy does not cause any immediate change in one's ability to function as, say, an amputation would, it might seem to be an easy adjustment. Some might even demean the importance of a breast. Some say that the breast is relatively useless anyway, especially once childbirth is completed.

A mastectomy is not just about survival, however. It is also about sexuality. The loss of a breast has an immediate and visible impact on one's sense of sexuality. Though the aging process inexorably lessens the sense of sexuality through a gradual loss of vitality and physical integrity, a mastectomy is a perceptible, immediate, irreversible blow to the self. It is true that youth is more vulnerable to these changes, yet sexuality is so central to our identity so as to transcend age. The author emphasizes how, in her experience as a middle-aged cancer survivor, coping with sexuality is crucial to overcoming the divisive effects of a mastectomy.

As this book points out, one must first find the will to survive. The impact of breast cancer, as is true for all serious cancers, is an awakening of sorts. It penetrates through the previously comforting denial of death in which we normally live. To deal with this initial shock of pain, one must draw upon an inner desire to overcome. This is not as straightforward as one might believe. Freud has said that the drive for self-preservation is not distinct like the sexual drive. A cauldron of confusion is predicable. A woman has just lost a part of herself that plays a role in nature's ability to continue life and once may have provided nourishment. Despite feeling diminished, she must find the motivation to grow and go forward again.

A will to survive is vital when confronting the complex challenge of recapturing sexuality following a mastectomy. The breast has several important roles in human sexuality. Psychologically, the breast is a real or symbolic icon of the pleasurable experience of suckling that pervades both childhood and adult sexual development. Secondly, it is a symbol of sexual satisfaction as conjured up in the image of cuddling with the breast. Add to this, the breast's role in lovemaking as a primary organ of sexual pleasure. For some, the breast may also be coveted as anatomically beautiful. Thus, loss of a breast creates a monumental disruption in the ability to feel sexual.

On a deeper level, a lost breast diminishes a woman's inner sense of identity because sexuality is a central theme in self-development. Freud teaches that there are stages of sexual development, starting in infancy. They culminate with a psychic struggle called the Oedipus complex, which emphasizes that sexual attraction is vital to emotional well-being. Successful human development leads to the eventual inhibition and sublimation of the sex drive. The redirected energy fuels the many pursuits of pleasure that both sustain us throughout our lives and motivate us to meet difficult demands. Having chosen survival over sexuality, the mastectomy patient is not able to draw upon this source of vitality. Attraction seems gone and may be replaced by repulsion and rejection; the inability to rival as demanded by oedipal conflicts may be experienced as extreme failure. The drive to pursue pleasure is stifled; a woman may not feel worthy of being desired sexually. Even the moral certainty of "doing the right thing" by having the operation does not help here, since attraction is not elevated by moral correctness. To the contrary, a certain "naughtiness" is more prone to elevate a sense of sexuality.

Besides the internal psychological struggles, for many there is a social impact to contend with following a mastectomy. With advances in the sophisticated technology of modern society, wide exposure is given to symbols of sexual perfection, resulting in the individual feeling society's ever greater demands to conform to exacting standards of sexuality. Today's mastectomy patient often has feelings of intense failure or humiliation in relation to the current social ideals. These feelings are intensified with the fear of unwanted discovery, since privacy seems harder to maintain in this age of information.

In *Mama Said There'd Be Days Like This*, the author concludes that one must work toward feeling whole again. A woman will never feel that others will accept her following a mastectomy until she has learned to fully accept herself. To those who are psychologically minded, the author offers the kind of guidance one will find invaluable in this lonely quest. My advice is, take your time, go slowly. Though this manual is short, the work of overcoming the effects of breast cancer and a mastectomy is not. To successfully resolve these issues may take years. Like the twelve steps of

Alcoholics Anonymous, a series of guiding principles and exercises can help you overcome something for which there is no formula. It can work if you try.

Peter Sugerman, M.D.

# AUTHOR'S NOTE

Both before and after undergoing a double mastectomy at the age of 47, I received many warm words of encouragement from women who had had this operation. They reached out to me, a stranger, and I will be forever grateful for their kindness. Still, I yearned to know **how** other women had struggled and come to terms with losing their breasts. How had they handled the intense feelings of fear, loss and humiliation that threatened to overwhelm me? How had they learned to accept a different body? I feel that having this type of knowledge as early as possible might have helped me get my bearings during what was a psychologically painful and disorienting time.

Left to my own resources, I could not prepare sufficiently for the emotional aftermath of the operation. I was sinking in psychological quicksand. I was afraid that if I let myself slip under the surface that I would lose my sanity. Losing part of my body was so different from anything I had experienced. Trying not to panic, I worked hard to visualize my goal. I would learn to think whatever I needed to think in order to feel normal and good again. One by one, I identified specific issues that were troubling me and developed strategies that allowed me to take a positive view of myself while dealing with those issues. Taking an active role was an important part of my healing process.

This book is divided into twelve steps that closely parallel my experience. In reality, however, the progression was not entirely linear. Rather, many thoughts and feelings were experienced simultaneously, and many issues had to be revisited repeatedly until they were resolved.

Although ultimately each of us heals uniquely, I often wished for a guide. Because there was no guide for me, I wrote this one for you.

## ACKNOWLEDGMENTS

This book has profited from the encouragement, feedback, and editing skills of the people kind enough to read it – in airplanes, in parking lots, at sporting events, and at kitchen tables. I would like to thank: Dorothy Benko, Beth Bruno, Karla Lee, Amy Kligerman, Laurie Kritzer, Dr. Lester Kritzer, Dr. Catherine Mermelstein, Dr. Peter Sugerman, Teri Swigut, Adam Smith, and Deby Vanohlen for their time and valuable perspectives, and also Sharon Friedlich, Esq. for sharing her legal expertise. A special thank-you goes to The J.M. Smucker Company for giving me permission to use their slogan in this book.

# CHOOSE LIFE

*"If I am not for myself, who will be for me?"*
—*Hillel*

    To have cancer is to become intimately acquainted with your own mortality. If you didn't before, you now know the fragility of life. Everyone and everything you love comes clearly into view. There are so many things you still want to experience and accomplish. Although it is true that we need a strong will to survive every day of our lives, it is when we are faced with a particularly threatening circumstance that we become acutely aware of our inner life force and our need to keep its flame strong.
    It is because we want to live so badly that we will do almost anything to give ourselves the best chance we can to survive. Giving up a breast, or two, is certainly an act of total desperation. Like an animal caught in a hunter's trap, we sacrifice part of the body in return for a chance to live. When people see an animal that has freed itself from a snare, they are perhaps put off at first by its appearance. Still, there is also a respect for the animal's inner strength and its will to survive.
    Do not let a mastectomy take away the life that you are fighting to save. The loss of part of your body is a great enough loss to suffer. Don't let it take away your dignity, your joy, your sexuality, or your sense of humor. Choose to live the rest of your life fully. Choose to live it as a whole person. Remember, mama said there'd be days like this.

However, with the help of a host of medical specialists and the support of your friends and family, you can get yourself through this. Make a commitment to do what it takes to make this tough adjustment. Believe that you can do it. Give it everything you've got because when you ask yourself just what you have to lose if you don't, you will find that the answer is — everything.

> *To survive, you must choose to live. At the same time, accept that there will be both bad and good times during the course of a life. Don't let the bad times cast a shadow over the good ones forever. Grieve and come to terms with painful events so that you can enjoy all the good things that you do have.*

# EXERCISE SET – 1

1. **Think Of People You Love.**

    *Make a list of all the people you love and try to spend time with them.*

2. **Think Of Things You Value.**

    *Make a list of all the things that mean the most to you and try to enjoy them.*

## 3. Think Of Your Goals.

*Make a list of all the things, big and small, that you still want to do and start to do them.*

## 4. Learn To Live In The Moment.

*Appreciate that with a heightened sense of the fragility of life, you are more able to live in the moment. Enjoy all the seemingly mundane things which are easy to take for granted.*

## 4. Have A Tug-Of-War.

Imagine drawing a line in the sand, and having a tug-of-war against Breast Cancer. Don't give Cancer any more than is absolutely necessary. You have lost one or both breasts. Concentrate on pulling on that rope and not letting Cancer get one more thing from you.

## 5. Do The Impossible.

Imagine doing something that seems impossible. In my mind, I would sometimes practice jumping over the Grand Canyon in one amazing leap. At other times, I might visualize going over the top of a tidal wave. It doesn't matter what scenario you choose. What is important is that you begin to see yourself doing something that you would have thought impossible. You can give yourself the message that even though you are facing a very challenging life circumstance, you can do what is necessary to help yourself through it.

# *HOUSTON, WE HAVE A PROBLEM*

*"There is more wisdom in your body than in your deepest philosophy."*
—Friedrich Nietzsche

Losing part of your body is a large threat to your emotional and mental well-being. It feels as if you have been caught in the headlights and the truck is heading straight at you. You are in danger. You are frightened. Still, it is in your best interest to put yourself into your own NASA-like control room and take full responsibility for your mission to recover your health. You cannot afford to act like a victim, because a victim doesn't have the power to help anyone. It is **you** who ultimately must learn to solve the problem of how to feel good about your changed body. To accept this fact is a large and necessary step in the right direction.

Focus as much energy as you possibly can as soon as you can on making this adjustment. When you do so you can take advantage of:

1. Your own sense of urgency - it is strong *now*, close to the time of the mastectomy.
2. The support you are able to get from other people – you will receive the maximum amount of support *now*.

As time goes by, the immediacy of this problem lessens. Other problems and situations compete for attention. The attention given to this one is diluted. The process of adjustment is slowed.

Over time you are also likely to get weighed down by any negative feelings that you develop about your changed body. The more negative you feel and the longer you feel that way, the harder it will be to reverse the negative spiral of feelings and to replace them with positive ones. You do not want to give the negative feelings a chance to be reinforced. So, although it might seem harder to solve this adjustment problem quickly, it is rather like skating over thin ice. It is when you skate over thin ice quickly that you are most apt to cross the lake safely.

Although you will not at first see how you are ever going to accept your new body, trust that you will learn to do so by listening carefully to your own thoughts and feelings. Trust that deep inside of yourself, you know how to survive.

*Empower yourself by taking full responsibility for your own well-being.*

# EXERCISE SET – 2

1. **Be The Commander Of An Important Mission.**

   *Whether you like it or not, you are in charge of your own well-being and you need to figure out what to do. Although it is a rather overwhelming feeling, focus on the fact that you have a big problem and that you can't afford to do anything other than work on solving it.*

2. **Set Up Internal Lines Of Communication.**

   *Do things that help you focus on what you are feeling and thinking. You need to be able to make the best use of your own knowledge and judgment:*

   - *Breathe – learn some breathing techniques or just take some deep breaths*
   - *Pray*
   - *Practice Yoga*
   - *Meditate*
   - *Grieve*
   - *Listen to Music – you know what you want to hear*
   - *Drum – perhaps the rhythms help to connect us to our own heartbeat, and to the heartbeat of life itself.*

## 3. Set Up External Lines Of Communication.

*You need to connect with others and with nature. You need to be able to get support and information from others and your environment.*

- *Get the support of friends and family. This is so very important. Although you have to adjust to the mastectomy, a cheering section makes you feel so much less isolated. If friends feel uncomfortable because they are not sure what to do, sometimes it helps to give them specific suggestions as to how to help you. For instance, ask for a five-minute weekly phone call or for a humorous e-mail. These small acts of kindness make you feel included in the life around you.*

  *Stay away from toxic people. You don't need people who treat you as an object of their pity, or are in other ways insensitive to your feelings. There are so many people who are compassionate. Spend your time with them.*

- *Physically connect with others through touch. Massage, professional or not, helps you feel better. Hugs and other affectionate forms of touch make you feel that others care.*

- *Commune with nature. Take a walk. Look around you. Feeling like part of the world, as opposed to apart from it, is healing.*

- *Share jokes and humorous stories. This helps you to see things in a new light.*

## 4. Connect With Your Inner Self.

*Connect with the part of yourself that you mean when you say "me". This is the part of you that does not change. This is the part of yourself that will, if you listen, tell you what you need to do.*

# *THE EYE OF THE TIGER*

*Let's roll!*

You will need to learn to deal with feelings of fear and terror that seem unending. When you do, you will be better able to help yourself both before and after surgery. Panic will block you from finding solutions to problems that you might otherwise have found. Indeed, people have drowned in situations in which they could have saved themselves had they not allowed panic to overtake them. Use your fear as a guide that is warning you about a great danger. Feeling the fear without letting it paralyze you helps you to protect yourself. You are better able to size up the danger with which you are faced and to take action in your own behalf.

One way I handled fear was to use my imagination to transform myself. In the same way that sports teams choose a symbol or team name such as "The Tigers," I found that I could identify with an animal that had a particular trait that I needed and "become" that animal. I found that I didn't have to limit myself to just one animal; I could use whatever image I needed at a given moment in order to "absorb" the characteristic that I wanted to possess.

I learned to understand the uses of masks, totems, and war paint in a whole new way. Instead of seeing them as strange things used in different cultures, I saw them as vehicles to help people become something more than they felt they were when it was just too scary to be their everyday, ordinary selves. Although I considered showing up for surgery in full war paint, I decided to do something a little more discreet. I went for a pedicure, and had my toenails painted bright red. That way, when they pushed me down that hall toward the surgical amphitheater, I had ten little badges of courage. I would need them all.

*Learn to use fear as a guide that alerts you to the dangers with which you are faced. You need to recognize that you are in danger and understand what the danger is before you can take action to protect yourself.*

# EXERCISE SET-3

1. **Nurture The Calm Strength Within You.**

    *You can use:*
    - *Breathing and relaxation techniques*
    - *Massage*
    - *Reiki – a technique that uses healing touch*
    - *Meditation*
    - *Visualization – visualize a positive outcome to your surgery.*

2. **Make Yourself Part Of Your Medical Team.**

    *Give yourself a job to do. OK, it won't be a well paying job; but when you have something to do it is easier not to give in to panic. Perhaps your job can be to keep the patient as calm as possible.*

3. **Desensitize Yourself.**

    *Desensitize yourself by looking at pictures of women with mastectomies. Try to take away the fear of the unknown.*

## 4. Minimize The Situation.

*If you are having reconstructive surgery done, you can imagine that one surgeon is going to take stuffing out of you and another is going to put the stuffing back. You can be like the straw man in "The Wizard of Oz."*

## 5. Imagine Doing Something Scary.

*Imagine doing something that scares you even more than the idea of your upcoming surgery. Visualize finding someone with a brand new driver's permit and volunteering to be the passenger. This will take your mind off things, at least for a few minutes.*

## 6. Face A Firing Squad.

*Before surgery, pretend you have to face a firing squad, and there is no escape. Although this visualization is not especially flattering to your doctors, it gives you the chance to practice keeping your dignity and personal power when faced with a situation in which you can easily lose them.*

## 7. To Everything There Is A Season.

*Take the drugs your doctor prescribes.*

## PIKES PEAK OR BUST

*"Reality, what a concept!"*
—Woody Allen

One method you can use to control your emotional pain deserves some special attention. You can start to become more aware of your thoughts. When you are feeling overwhelmed by anguish you can learn to focus totally on something about which you have positive feelings. When you totally focus on one image, you will find that you have effectively blocked all other images from your mind. It is a great relief to learn that you can only focus deeply on one thing at a time, and that you can choose the image. When you control your thoughts you also control the associated feelings. You have control over how you experience your world.

If you take this concept a step farther, you can see that we are always selectively paying attention to parts of our world. What we see depends on how we look at it. What we call reality is therefore not a static thing. Our reality is always being redefined by our perception. This opens the possibility of changing your present view of reality concerning the loss of a breast. Although you can't change the fact that a breast has been lost, you can learn to choose your thoughts, and therefore your feelings, about this event. You can realize that you have always selected your view of reality.

*Learn that although we cannot always choose our circumstances, we do have control over our responses to them.*

*Karen Klein*

# EXERCISE SET-4

### 1. The White Spot.

- *Imagine a black piece of paper with a tiny white spot on it.*

- *Learn to focus totally on the white spot so that it is the only thing that you can see.*

- *Then visualize the black piece of paper again. This time make the white spot a bit bigger than before. Again, focus totally on the white spot.*

- *Continue this exercise, varying the size of the white spot.*

- *Make the white spot so large it fills the paper until there is only a tiny speck of black left. Continue to focus on the white area.*

*What you want to learn from this exercise is that it doesn't matter how small or large the white area is. If you are totally focusing on the white spot, you will see white. When you are focusing on the white spot, it doesn't really matter how large the black area is. You will still be experiencing the white spot.*

## 2. Focus on the Positive.

*Realize that at any given moment you can choose to focus on the positive or the negative aspects of an event. What you choose to focus on is your experience. You can choose the white spot no matter how small or how large it is. Although you are in a more extreme situation than usual, you are always choosing your perception. By choosing how you experience an event, you are also choosing how you will feel about the event.*

## 3. Question What You Know.

*Before Christopher Columbus sailed to the New World, most people in Europe thought the earth was flat. Since Columbus's journey, most people think it is round. Is it possible that other experiences will one day teach us to envision the earth in yet another way? Can we really know the shape of the earth, or are we always just working with our best picture of it?*

*Just like Columbus, we must keep our minds open and explore new ways of looking at the world. What we think of as a fact may be only our best guess at the present time. We can learn to be explorers with bold and original visions that will allow us to do new and exciting things. Like Columbus, we can look at something old in a new way. We can look at our altered bodies and choose to see that new possibilities may be just beyond the horizon.*

# "A" IS FOR ADAPTING

*"When you come to a fork in the road, take it."*
—Yogi Berra

You need to adapt to an unwanted change. This is hard enough to do without compounding your problem by allowing yourself to internalize a negative self-image. Now, more than ever, you need to see yourself in a strong, positive light.

Following a mastectomy, it is common to have the following thinking pattern:

1. I saw myself as good (attractive, whole).
2. I do not see myself as good now.
3. How can I ever see myself as good again, since my body will always be different from now on?

The trouble with this mind-set is that if the only way you can see yourself as good again is to be the same as you were before, this is not going to happen. With or without plastic surgery your body will still be different from your pre-surgery body. Now, besides needing to make a difficult adjustment, you have to learn to feel "good" again, and you have labeled yourself as "bad."

Instead, choose to think:

1. I saw myself as good (attractive, whole).
2. I see myself as good now.
3. I will see myself as good in the future.

Realize that you change every day; you age, for example. In many ways you never go back to the way you were before – not only physically, but also mentally and emotionally. Change is a part of life and you always need to adapt to it. So, if you look at a mastectomy as a change that requires you to adjust, you have a very challenging problem. However, this is a solvable problem and it is one with which you already have some experience.

You need to adapt to a different body. Still, you can preserve and even strengthen a positive self-image. To this end, focus on images that make you feel good about yourself. Even though you have no idea how you will ever really see yourself as beautiful or how you will come to terms with your altered body, do not allow yourself to focus on negative images of yourself. Find something about yourself that you like and focus on it. Whether you choose to think about your beautiful legs, your artistic ability, or your fighting spirit, the important thing is to continue to experience yourself in a positive way. The more you can keep a positive self-image, the more energy you will have available to learn to adapt to this change. Besides, when you feel good about yourself, you feel good.

*Learn to adapt to changing circumstances while staying connected to the part of you that has not changed. Consider that if you were in a poker game, being dealt a good hand would not make you "good", and being dealt a bad hand would not make you "bad". How you define yourself needs to be based on something more enduring than changing circumstances.*

# EXERCISE SET-5

1. **Draw On Your Own Experience.**

   *Identify things in your life to which you have successfully adapted. Perhaps you have moved to a new school, a new house, or a new city. Perhaps you have changed jobs, marital status, or had children.*

   - *How did you deal with the changes that challenged you?*

   - *How did you feel before you had adjusted to the change?*

   - *What did you do to cope with your feelings?*

   - *What did you do to help yourself adjust to your new situation?*

   - *How did you feel after you were adjusted to the change?*

   *You can draw on your own experience to find the kinds of actions that will help you adapt.*


2. **Visualize Yourself Coping Successfully With Unwanted Changes.**

   *Imagine some change in your life that would be distressing to you. It doesn't matter how silly it is.*

   - *Someone comes to your house and takes away all the furniture you have taken years to save up for, and replaces it with a style you totally hate.*

- Someone grabs you, pulls you into the bushes, and gives you the most terrible haircut that anyone has ever had. They then dump you on your front lawn. Oh, I forgot to tell you ... you're getting married tomorrow!

Visualize how you would deal successfully with these situations. It is important to see yourself coping well with unwanted change. You need to see yourself as coming out on top in a situation where your first trillion wishes are not going to come true.

### 3. Ride A Bucking Bronco.

In this exercise, you need to visualize yourself in a dangerous and new situation. Perhaps you have landed on a bucking bronco. Realize that this isn't the time to ponder whether or not you would like to sign up for bronco riding lessons. You are on the bronco right now. Focus on learning to be the best bucking bronco rider that ever existed. Make this a priority. Figure out how to ride right now.

### 4. Laughing Out Loud.

Finding the humor in a difficult situation helps you adapt by finding new ways to look at what you are experiencing. Besides, laughing out loud also causes your body to make endorphins, chemicals that help to strengthen your immune system. Sometimes when things are so bad, you just have to laugh.

## THE WISE WARRIOR WOMAN

*"We are what we pretend to be..."*
—Kurt Vonnegut

Losing one or both breasts is hard to adapt to partly because we consider it to be a negative change. It wouldn't be as difficult to accept if, as a society, we thought it was a desirable look. I realize that we don't think that, and that probably no other civilization on the planet does either. Still, there are many cultures that scar, stretch, or otherwise mutilate the human body, often to beautify it in their eyes. These practices may seem strange and even repulsive to people outside a particular culture. They are, however, accepted in a certain context.

We consider the loss of breasts to be negative because, in the context of our culture it is negative. I needed, then, to find a context in which I could accept such a change, even if no one else could or would. Although many women have had to adjust to mastectomies, I was the one who now had to find a way to look at this "disfigurement" in a new way. To this end I set up a "theater of the mind." It was entirely in my imagination. I pictured a movie screen and even used my thumb to push an imaginary button to change "slides." With practice, I could even zoom in and out to crop pictures. I was concentrating on finding suitable images that might help me accept having no breasts, so although I viewed thousands of images, the search was not entirely willy-nilly. My mind helped me to close in on some helpful images, and your mind will help you.

The image that first helped me was that of a wise warrior woman. If there was a secret tribe of wise warrior women, similar to the mythical Amazon women, who chose to have no breasts and I was one of them – then I would be able to feel good about myself when I was with them. I decided that I would turn myself into a wise warrior woman. I would transform myself. I would be able to feel good about my body. I did, too. For about forty minutes one morning I was a member of a secret sect of wise warrior women. While it was somewhat embarrassing, even in the confines of my own mind, it was an important private victory. I had learned to work with images and put them in different contexts to gain control over how I looked at things. I had taken some control over this situation, and with practice I could gain more.

By engaging in similar visualizations, you can develop the flexibility of thought necessary to adapt. You will not be trapped or limited by one mind-set. Think outside the box. If one way of looking at things is not working for you, free yourself to find another.

*Free yourself from the constraints of time and place by looking at your circumstances in different contexts.*

## EXERCISE SET-6

### Remember the Ugly Duckling.

Keep looking for contexts in which you can accept your new body. It doesn't matter how unrealistic they are. The thought process itself will move you toward resolution and acceptance.

**The Ugly Duckling** can always be used as the basis of your visualizations. We all know that the ugly duckling is really a beautiful swan. Concentrate on being that swan. Hold your head high on that long, graceful neck. You will feel as if you are in a very large pond, chock-full of those darned ducks. Rest assured that every duck has its day.

# THE POLLYANNA PRINCIPLE

*"People are about as happy as they make up their minds to be."*
—Abraham Lincoln

Having a mastectomy is extremely painful partly because of the magnitude of the change experienced within a short time span. Change, both positive and negative, is stressful. A death in the family is stressful, but so is a marriage or the birth of a baby. We don't like things to be too much the same, either. We enjoy a certain rate of change that feels comfortable to us. So, I thought, if my chest had gotten flat very slowly over enough time, I would have experienced a series of micro losses and micro adjustments. Although this would not have been experienced as a good thing, it would not have been as traumatic either. Change occurs in our lives every day, and we handle it.

To see this change, mastectomies, as an extreme case of a familiar situation allowed me to feel some control again. Looking at the process of aging, we know that we age every day. Having a mastectomy is like waking up and finding that you are fifty years older after only one day. It is shocking in that it is rather more than we usually have to bear at one time. Still, when you look at a lifetime of aging, you can see both a long line of losses and a long line of gains. This is why at forty you can look back at how you were at twenty and still feel that you have come out fine when everything is taken into account. You know that you have lost in some areas but have gained in others.

While suffering from a great loss, I needed to grieve, but I also needed to learn how to strengthen the part of the process that finds the positives in the present situation. Pollyanna, we remember from the Disney movie, plays the "Glad Game," finding the good in everything and everyone around her. Finding and celebrating everything that is positive, including things about your new body shape, will help you to adapt. This is asking a lot of a person, to be sure. However, I believed it was in my own best interest to become the quintessential "Glad Game" player. To that end, I learned to be so positive I would have made that Pollyanna girl puke.

What could possibly be positive about having both breasts replaced with saline implants?

1. My breasts would be permanently perky.
2. It would be a lot easier to get into a cold swimming pool.
3. I would rarely need a bra.
4. I would not need a mammogram.
5. During a full moon, I would be able to experience high tide.

The power of positive thinking is that it leads to positive action. Although you have to let go of the old, you discover new possibilities. In the short run, however, it is necessary to go around and pound on a lot of doors to find out which ones will open.

*Give yourself hope for your future by focusing on the positives of your situation.*

## EXERCISE SET-7

### 1. Celebrate Everything That Is Positive.

*List anything that has been positive about your mastectomy experience. Perhaps you have become closer to certain friends or family members. Maybe you now feel more compassion for people. Maybe you can more easily squeeze into the space between the car and the garage wall.*

### 2. Run A Lemonade Stand.

*You are running a lemonade company; your supplier has just delivered a huge load of oranges and has driven away. You have to produce enough lemonade by tomorrow morning to fill your orders or else you will not make enough money to pay the rent. You must make this situation work in order for your business to survive.*

*To solve this problem, concentrate on identifying your strengths in the lemonade business. Come up with constructive things you can do to solve your problem. Call the marketing department. Figure out how to make orange flavored lemonade an acceptable substitute by tomorrow. Learn to focus on what you do have and what you can do. Positive thinking will help you to strengthen the habits required to optimize every available avenue of action.*

*Practice finding the smallest positive aspects of a situation that you can and visualizing the positive actions that would lead to a successful conclusion.*

## 3. Learn To Let Go.

*While you are learning to emphasize the positives of your new body, you also have to let go of the old one. To that end, practice the art of letting go of things:*

- *Breathe, and concentrate on exhaling.*

- *If people say irritating things, let them roll off your back. This is a good skill to practice at holiday gatherings.*

- *Clean out closets and let go of the old unused items.*

- *Forgive others. Let go of bad feelings.*

# MIRROR, MIRROR

*"No one can make you feel inferior
without your permission."*
—Eleanor Roosevelt

When you look in the mirror what do you see? A woman with a mastectomy may see a mutilated woman who will forever be devalued by society. A teenager with a pimple on her nose may see an ugly girl who might as well not go to the party. A model may focus on the dimple of cellulite on her thigh and feel washed-up. A woman of a certain age may see a face full of wrinkles and feel unattractive. All these people have something in common. They need a new mirror.

I once had the opportunity to hear a man who had been born with a non-traditional body speak about his life. He wore two artificial legs and had still learned to play tennis. His hands were also unconventionally shaped. He spoke about how in kindergarten, as part of an art project, the children in the class were supposed to put their handprints on their papers. He was concerned, understandably, about how his handprint would look to the other children. His teacher, however, was sensitive and told him that she valued all of her students' work. This statement helped him change his perception of himself. He saw himself as a student. His hand was the hand of a student. He went on to discuss other challenges he had faced in his life. By the end of the talk, those listening to him saw him as someone to whom they could relate. Since he presented himself in a dignified and personable way, people reacted well to him. At the conclusion of his presentation, everyone stood in line to shake his hand.

The actress, Marlee Matlin, is another great role model for those who see themselves as being "different." Although she is hearing impaired, she has appeared in many television programs, including "The West Wing." She is attractive, intelligent and accomplished. It is not difficult to imagine that many attractive, intelligent and accomplished people would be drawn to her. Since she does not see herself as "less," neither do we. She does not define herself as "the deaf girl," thereby emphasizing what is different about her. She defines herself in ways that allow others to see many aspects of her self. People notice that she cannot hear as well as they can, but that is only part of her identity.

We must make a choice. We can consider ourselves to be damaged and play the part of the victim. When we do that, in effect, we are choosing to relegate ourselves to a street corner like the proverbial blind man holding a tin cup. We can choose instead to see ourselves as mountain climbers who simply don't see as well as others. Erik Weihenmayer was the first blind climber to make it to the top of Mount Everest. If he had chosen to stand on a street corner he would not have been able to enjoy his spectacular triumph.

Although how we see ourselves is a reflection of how others see us, other people also see us as we see ourselves. It has been said that people take us at our own estimation; in other words, we teach others how to treat us. This is true for everyone, even those with all their original body parts. We must all define ourselves. It is the difference between being a gray puff or a gray panther, between being a loser or a winner in the making, between being a gimpy woman or a woman full of grace. You are always you no matter how you change, and when you concentrate on all that is beautiful, both your mirror and your world will reflect that, beautifully.

*To a great degree, the quality of our lives is determined by how we see ourselves. Learn that you have the power to influence your self-image. Do not give that power away.*

*Karen Klein*

# EXERCISE SET-8

1. **Climb Mount Everest.**

    *Choose to model yourself after people like Marlee Matlin or Erik Weihenmayer. See yourself as a person who pursues her goals and learns to overcome any and all obstacles. The goal here is to visualize succeeding at something new and challenging. Perhaps you will choose to climb Mount Everest. Close your eyes and see yourself climbing, focusing on your goal, and never giving up. Make sure that you see yourself making it all the way to the top.*

2. **Learn To Avoid Self-Pity.**

    *Play the game you can call "Do Not Go To The Corner. Do Not Pick Up The Cup." The object of this very serious game is not to become a victim of self-pity. There is nothing easy about this. It is a huge challenge, but if you made it up Mount Everest you have the stamina to do what is necessary to win this game.*

    *Here is how you play: whenever you start to feel sorry for yourself, say either aloud or silently, "I will not go to the corner. I will not pick up the cup." Then quickly "become" a mountain climber, start to climb a mountain, and say, "I choose to be a mountain climber. I choose to climb the mountain." Focus and remain focused on getting to the mountaintop. By doing this, you are training yourself to replace negative feelings with positive ones. Feel proud that you are helping yourself by taking a positive mental course of action. When you stand at the mountain's peak, wave that flag.*

*Mama Said There'd Be Days Like This*

You are allowed to feel sad, grieve, and cry freely. What you cannot do, however, is to see yourself on a corner, cup in hand. You are not to imagine that you need to be pitied. If you devalue yourself in any way, you lose a round of this game. It's OK, just don't give up. Try again, and feel good about keeping up your efforts.

Keep in mind that spending time with people who pity you undermines the hard work you are doing to keep from pitying yourself. Pity is destructive to your self-esteem. It is degrading. Do the best you can to avoid such people.

### 3. The Diamond.

You might want to try another way to resist the psychological pressure to see yourself as having less worth than you did before your surgery. In this visualization, let yourself feel the pressure in all of its raw fury. Feel as if you are in a crucible and that the pressure will either crush you or turn you into a magnificent diamond. By now you know to choose to visualize letting the searing heat and unbearable pressure form you into that diamond.

### 4. Tiara Times.

Sometimes, to remind yourself just how beautiful you are, you might choose to wear a tiara. I chose to keep this an "at home" activity, but you may choose differently.

## *PLAN B*

*With a name like Smucker's, it has to be good.® ***
—The J.M. Smucker Company

    Although I had never wanted to be a Cosmo cover girl before undergoing a double mastectomy, there was something about feeling that the possibility had disappeared forever that made me weep. Despite all my positive thinking was I, in the end, going to feel "damaged?" Was I, in reality, stuck in a losing situation? I needed to look at things from yet another angle. I decided that in addition to learning to redefine myself, I would also try to see how I could take a fresh look at the definition of beauty.
    Scientists have looked at what people in different cultures find beautiful when looking at another person. They have found that symmetry is important. Also, the various features found to be beautiful are mathematically proportionate to each another. The researchers think that the reason symmetrical, well-proportioned people are found to be beautiful and desirable is that these properties signal good health. If you choose to mate with someone with good health, there is a greater chance that you and your children will be healthy and survive. Having characteristics that make you more likely to survive and thrive in your environment makes you attractive.

---

* *Used with the permission of The J.M. Smucker Company.*

So, losing part of my body definitely wasn't helping me to put myself together and present myself as a healthy survival package. Having cancer wasn't helping either. How could this situation be so bad in so many ways? How could I still see myself as whole and beautiful? I didn't know, but I did know a few things.

1. There would be no reward for giving up on this problem.
2. A belief that no one would want me could easily become a self-fulfilling prophecy.
3. If I sank into a pool of self-pity then even I wouldn't want me.
4. I would need to keep the most important vote, my own, and consider every vote after that to be a bonus.
5. No one likes a whiner, even if she does have great breasts.

If adapting to your environment and surviving is what ultimately makes you attractive, then we can question anew which "looks" can be considered beautiful. To be adaptable is now to be beautiful, and all the forms of existing life are beautiful in their own way. A frog is beautiful, a cat is beautiful, and a person is beautiful. We can now look at the relationship between survival and beauty in a new way.

At first, we put the focus on looking pretty in a way accepted by our culture, because looking pretty is valued and has helped us to survive. Now we can, instead, put the focus more directly on our ability to adapt. We can do this when we recognize that this is the larger, all-encompassing trait that ultimately has the most survival value for us. Since it has the most survival value, it is our ability to adapt that makes us beautiful.

We need to learn to appreciate the many forms life

takes and be able to appreciate that we were one form and are now another of these beautiful forms. It is our ability to change when we need to that makes us beautiful. The better we become at adapting, the more beautiful we become. To this end, we can learn to use our imaginations and to "morph" from one beautiful form to another. You want to develop this skill so that you are able to imagine yourself starting out as one thing and turning into another. You want to imagine you are beautiful in all your various forms. This will help you learn to feel more comfortable with the changed shape of your body. It takes a lot of concentration and energy. If you get tired and need a break, you can always curl up in a cocoon and take a nap before you turn yourself into a beautiful butterfly.

*Learn to differentiate between timeless beauty and current style.*

*Karen Klein*

# EXERCISE SET-9

### 1. Learn To Morph.

Visualize "morphing" from one life form to another to yet another. See yourself changing from one animal or person to another. Perhaps you will see yourself first as a baby, then as a young girl, and finally as a woman. Perhaps you will see yourself as a fish, then a bear, and then an eagle. The goal here is to do this often enough to become used to having your outer appearance change. Try to make the transitions feel fluid. Concentrate on learning to feel comfortable in whatever form you take. When you do, the changes will feel less frightening. This exercise will help train you to feel comfortable with the changes in your body.

### 2. Appreciate Different Styles.

Visualize having a work of art and having it change into another work of art. Perhaps you will start off with a Rubens and end up with a Picasso. Both are highly valued pieces of art. They are just different styles. Concentrate on learning to appreciate the new style. Think of yourself as getting more sophisticated. You have an acquired taste. You can think whatever you want to as long as you think that each one is good.

### 3. Become A Good Marketer.

As a woman, you will understand the idea of changing negative associations with positive ones by the way we learn to accept new fashion trends. One season we will be wearing pants that we wouldn't even have considered wearing one short season ago. How do the marketers do it? They link the image of a woman wearing weird pants with something that we consider positive. You can do the same thing with your body. Feel encouraged. Be a good marketer. Just remember – it's not purple, it's "eggplant" and it's not weird, it's "haute-couture." Sell your body to yourself. Train yourself to think differently about your body. It is difficult, but the reward is a big one. You can feel good again.

### 4. Dare To Be Different.

*Sometimes a different strategy can be helpful. Start a "Dare to be Different" club and run for president. Allow yourself to enjoy your different body and to be happy about it, without feeling the least bit apologetic. Adopt an "in your face" attitude. This feels really good for a change, doesn't it?*

## NIPPLES OPTIONAL

*"Who are those guys?"*
—from *"Butch Cassidy and the Sundance Kid"*

Many women choose not to have plastic surgery after a mastectomy. For those who do, there are several techniques by which the surgeon is able to create "breasts." I chose to have saline implants, but no matter what you decide, I think that it is helpful if in your own mind you ask:

1. What can a plastic surgeon do for me?
2. What will I have to do for myself?

Before answering these questions, it is necessary to consider your ideas about self-esteem. I believe that it is useful to recognize two different types of self-esteem.

The first type is social self-esteem. In this type of self-esteem your sense of self-worth is tied to how others value you. A fancy car, the right address, or a beautiful body might make you feel good because you feel more valued when you have such things. When you don't or can't have what is acceptable in your social group, you will have a sense of reduced self-esteem.

The second type of self-esteem is individual self-esteem. It is based on your own evaluation of your self-worth, independent of your social group's opinion. It is based, instead, on your own inner value system. When you place individual self-esteem above social self-esteem, you are better able to take an unpopular stand. A solid sense of individual self-esteem allows you to say "no" to drugs, become a dancer instead of a doctor, or become a doctor when no one in your neighborhood thinks school is cool. Rosa Parks showed her strong sense of individual self-esteem when she refused to give up her seat on the bus. This type of self-esteem can't be bought, sewed in, bleached out, or chopped off you. It can only be earned by developing your own inner fortitude. If you can stand up for yourself using your individual self-esteem you may not always have the goodies, but you will definitely always have the goods.

What then can a plastic surgeon do for you? If you are lucky, a good plastic surgeon can provide you with a good, built-in breast prosthesis. It does not, in my opinion, give you back a breast. Still, if you want a more traditional adult female shape and find it preferable to a prosthesis that you wear outside your body, this type of surgery can be a very wonderful option. Whether you feel better with an artificial breast or none at all depends partly on your personal sensibilities and partly on the results of your surgery.

If you are looking for social self-esteem, I think reconstructed breasts have value, but the value is limited. The emphasis remains on getting the breasts back, and this is not possible. Surgically constructed breasts are different from natural breasts, and the difference will always be experienced as a loss. If you develop your individual self-esteem, however, surgery can still provide only a partial solution, but it is a workable one. You more easily give up the expectation that the new breasts will replace the original ones. You are then better able to grieve your loss totally and to accept that your body will be different than it was, forever. This frees you to consider the reconstructed breasts as different, but to appreciate them for what they are and what they can give you. You are in a compromise situation. Take the compromise.

*Learn to differentiate between self-image and body- (or social) image.*

*Karen Klein*

# EXERCISE SET-10

## 1. Ride With Rosa.

Be inspired by Rosa Parks; feel equal to others and entitled to your dignity. Picture yourself refusing to give up your seat on a bus when everyone else expects you to stand. You will realize how difficult it is to do something all alone, without support. However, if you learn to keep your seat on this bus, you will have earned enough self-esteem to last you a lifetime.

While sitting on that bus you can:

- Imagine that your skeleton is made of titanium.

- Imagine that the universe is roaring at you and you are roaring back.

- Imagine drinking a few gallons of testosterone.

## 2. Bond With Your Body.

When I first got my saline implants, it was very odd to have something foreign in my body. I thought I could consider the implants to be aliens from a distant planet. My plan was to try to co-exist with them in peace.

In a very short time, I realized that I would feel better if I accepted the aliens and made them a part of me. Still, they were so different from my old breasts! What had I been thinking when I agreed to have implants? Had I made a foolish choice because I had felt so desperate? I felt naïve for hoping that a doctor could fix me. I was embarrassed. I had never even gotten a good idea of what the implants would look like before I agreed to get them. This lack of knowledge had made it impossible to prepare myself for the reality of what my reconstructed breast would be like. I felt blindsided. Despite all that surgery, I would still have a huge adjustment to make.

Since I was too embarrassed to ask my doctor to take the implants out, I began to look for ways to get used to them. Once again, I tried to see how I could make the unfamiliar seem more comfortable to me.

These breasts were very hard. Well — my breasts had been hard when they had been engorged with milk. I could pretend that they were now similarly engorged. This time, however, the engorgement would never go away. Still, I had coped with hard breasts before. I could do it again.

These breasts had no feeling in them. I tried to imagine that I had lost feeling in them over time. They were now just somewhat less sensitive than they had been previously.

It was easier for me to accept a new situation by finding the parts of it that seemed familiar. You can use the same technique if you had a surgical procedure different from mine, or had no surgery at all. One way or another, you will have to cope with a large change in your body image.

## 3. Go Faux.

To get used to man-made breasts, celebrate all that is man-made. Get faux nails, faux hair or dyed hair, faux jewels, and faux animal skin clothing. Realize that these things are good things. Enjoy them.

## 4. Practice Makes Imperfect.

*Practice feeling OK about being relatively unskilled at a new activity. For instance, I decided to try my hand at golf and joined a league. On the first day, my score was 117 – for nine holes! What was important was that I had the chance to practice dealing with a situation in which I was not measuring up to an ideal image. I was able to experience that no real disaster followed my poor round of golf. Other people's reactions to my poor skill level were, to a large extent, based on mine. Since I could laugh at myself, they laughed with me, not at me. The next week, the golf pro told me that he admired me for coming back. Sometimes it is all about coming back.*

## SAVE THE LAST DANCE

*"Love is not love which alters
when it alteration finds."*
—William Shakespeare

Although the overwhelming temptation is to worry about how present or potential romantic partners will react to an altered body, you will be doing yourself a favor if you resist the urge to torture yourself with thoughts of eternal rejection. Trying to stave these feelings off is harder than saying "no" when the potato chips are being passed around. Could just one hurt? Yes, it could.

Will my husband (boyfriend, partner) feel differently about me after I have a mastectomy? Will they see me differently? How different will this part of my life be?

The answer is an individual one. It depends. As I have said in earlier sections, how you are seen is greatly dependent on how you see yourself and how you act. Also, how your partner reacts tells you a lot about their character. Do you really want someone who doesn't treat you very well at a time like this? Besides, accepting poor treatment sets you up to be treated poorly even if you are a high fashion model and considered to be very attractive. If you don't want to be treated like less, don't act like less.

While it is hard to deal with the change in the physical appearance of your own body, I still feel that:

- Taking control of the sexual part of your life and keeping it as normal as possible helps to keep life as normal as possible.

- This is a good opportunity to learn to become very poised. You'll be able to show up to a formal event in shorts and handle the situation well after this.

- You can feel fortunate; pretty much the only thing in life you have to do totally naked is take a shower.

- If the change in your body is making the idea of having sex uncomfortable, try to do something at first to help make the experience more familiar. It is the fear that things will be different that is so upsetting; try experiencing sex in a way that can seem as normal as possible. For instance, wearing a cute tee shirt and visualizing or having a series of "quickies" might help you to focus on that which can be the same.

Although keeping life as normal as possible is a good thing, you also have to allow yourself to pay attention to any negative feelings that you have, and to express and deal with them. For example, at one point I was concerned that I would not be attractive to other men. My husband wasn't thrilled, but he did agree to play the part of a stranger and pick me up in a bar. Although it might seem silly, this gave me something to do about my anxiety and fear. Giving myself an avenue of action helped me to feel in control. Consequently, it became easier to let go of the negative feelings. Approaching any problem during this whole process with some sense of power brought great relief.

After all is said and done, I think that at some time most of us have felt insecure in regard to some part of our bodies. There are the fat thighs, drooping breasts, and after-baby abdomens that challenge us to accept our bodies and not let negative feelings get in the way of enjoying our lives. A chest without breasts or with reconstructed breasts can be successfully dealt with employing the same strategies you have used with every other part of you that doesn't measure up to an imagined ideal. Besides, you can decide to use this time of your life as a wonderful opportunity to learn what you already know, that love and true caring have nothing to do with body parts. When you're on the dance floor with your partner and the music changes, you can begin a new dance together.

*Learn to trust that you are lovable regardless of external circumstances. You have intrinsic worth.*

Karen Klein

# EXERCISE SET-11

### 1. Ain't No River Wide Enough.

When you feel secure and good about yourself, you are able to consider someone else's negative evaluation of you as an opinion rather than a confirmation of a truth. You see what they say as statements that reflect who they are, rather than statements about you. The same is true of their actions. Not all partners, present or potential, can or will see past your chest wall and care for you as a person. This painful reality hurts. Still, if you lower your opinion of yourself, you will become less attractive to those who are willing and able to respond positively to the woman you are. While you can, perhaps, attract fewer partners, they are the ones who are more likely to stay with you and be supportive at times like these. After seeing just how tough life can be, don't you want a partner who can and will act as though there "ain't no river wide enough," rather than someone who is extremely worried about ruining their new shoes?

Practice being happy about being better able to separate the wheat from the chaff.

### 2. Rejection Fantasies.

If you feel you must have fantasies of people running from you and screaming in horror after viewing your body, do yourself one favor. Make sure that one really wonderful person remains after all the others have left. This person is just for you and is ready, willing, and able to be a part of your life. Remember that this is your fantasy. Why shouldn't you give it a happy ending?

### 3. Tender Loving Care.

*Give yourself a little extra TLC. If you don't do it now, when should you do it?*

- *Go to a spa or pamper yourself at home.*

- *Exercise, eat well, and try to get a good night's sleep.*

- *Take some extra time and effort with your appearance.*

- *Go shopping – get a new outfit, some new makeup, or a piece of jewelry.*

### 4. True Love.

*Finding you have a loving and accepting partner even when you are not feeling your best can lead to some very special moments. Cherish them.*

## THE BIG PICTURE

*"Why walk when you can fly?"*
—Mary Chapin Carpenter

What do you do when you have gotten to the end of the road, and you are not at your destination? How can you truly feel beautiful when your body will never be the way you really wish it would be? How, in the end, can you make the unacceptable acceptable?

What can we do when we can do no more? We are humbled by the fact that our bodies are broken and our minds are limited. Since we can do no more from our limited point of view, we must then learn to transcend our limitations by learning to look at life from a point of view without those limitations. Where the old road stops, we must begin to build a new road.

How can we reconcile inner beauty with outer beauty? In our usual way of thinking, they are two separate things. However, we can begin to look at the relationship between the inside and the outside. Where is the dividing line? Where is the end of the outside? Where is the beginning of the inside? We can begin to look at the whole as a continuum, and at the subdivisions of the whole as arbitrary. Instead of looking at day and night, we can focus on a twenty-four hour period as a unit. We can see that day and night are two ways of experiencing the same thing. Instead of focusing on spring, summer, fall, or winter, we can focus on the whole year. We can see that the subdivisions are again, arbitrary.

Working backward, we can fuse everything in the universe together as one, unified whole.

There are advantages to looking at things in this manner:

1. There is now a constant, coherent whole. Instead of experiencing things as being different, they just appear to be different depending on how you are looking at them.

2. Our greatest fear is the fear of the unknown. We feel that our survival is threatened. We don't know how to adapt to the unknown. This point of view makes everything known by making everything constant, even time. We are, therefore, always able to anchor ourselves to the familiar. Since we now know that we are seeing something familiar, but in an unfamiliar way, we can start to make sense of our new situation by seeing how it relates to our old, familiar one.

3. It is in the unified whole that we can recreate our reality. By tapping into the infinite possibilities of new ways of looking at things, finding new ways to fuse things together and new ways to subdivide them out again, we redefine our world. We can achieve a flexibility of thought that goes beyond the defined, arbitrary boundaries that made up our original mind-sets. Our viewpoint was limited, but by changing our point of reference to one that is outside of us, it no longer is. In that moment of recognition that we can do this, we begin to learn to fly. It is in this place of infinite possibilities that we can truly learn to adapt to new and challenging

circumstances.

4. Also, if the inside and outside of ourselves are arbitrary subdivisions of reality, then we can fuse them together and look at things differently. If we perceive a change either inside or outside of ourselves (it doesn't matter which because we look at them as a fused whole), we try to regain balance, or adapt.

Two things can happen:

- We can be in a maladaptive state in which we are either not attuned to the messages we are receiving that tell us we need to rebalance or we are unable to respond to them. If we are unable to receive the messages that change is necessary to rebalance, the messages persist, causing wear and tear on our minds and bodies.

- We can be in an adaptive state, able to rebalance and adapt, by being sensitive to the changes occurring in our environments (both inner and outer) and by allowing ourselves to make the adjustments necessary for our own well-being. When our thoughts, feelings, and actions are integrated and we are able to be both sensitive enough to perceive change and flexible enough to be able to rebalance, then we achieve a state of optimal health. In other words, optimal adaptability is optimal health. We still need to see that it is in this state of optimal adaptability and health that we experience optimal beauty.

As living beings, we have evolved with the help of our survival instincts. During times of great challenge, we are often more willing to listen to what we already know deep inside. We are drawn to that which is beautiful. It is, in fact, because something helps us to survive that we find it beautiful. It is when we experience the unity of the world, which we do through our own compassion and feelings of connection to everything, that we see the big picture. It is in the big picture that we feel the true beauty of the unity and of ourselves as a part of it. It is when we feel truly beautiful, that we are beautiful, truly.

*Learn to accept the seeming dual nature of the universe by experiencing its underlying unity.*

*Mama Said There'd Be Days Like This*

# EXERCISE SET-12

1. Learn From The Martial Arts.

When you are clearly not strong enough to beat your opponent, you can learn to take advantage of your opponent's strength. You can learn to use all the available energy in a situation, not just yours. Thinking about how to use all the power to your advantage may require you to change your mind-set. You can start by imagining some strategies that you might use if you were to engage in the martial arts.

2. Create Continuums.

Try to look at some seeming opposites differently. Look at an object and see the inside and outside as a continuum. If you start by considering the inside and then move toward the outside, each area is more outside and less inside than the previous area. Still, even when you reach the most outside area, you can consider that even that area is not purely outside.

When looking at joy and sorrow, you can fuse them into a continuum, or gradient. Even when you are at the joy end of the continuum it has some sorrow in it. The sorrow end of the continuum also has some joy. So, the elements of the fused whole are the same, it is just that the concentration of the elements in different areas of the continuum is different.

By viewing pairs as one unit, you can concentrate on what is the same about them. When you can identify the similarities, you can more easily adjust to the changed environment. This is because you no longer have to adapt to something that is totally different. Rather, your new situation contains the same elements as the old situation, only in different proportions.

Try imagining that you are a water animal that has to learn to live in the air. Try to imagine a water to air continuum. Start off on the water end. Now move to the next area that is a little less water and a little more air. Can you get used to living here? It is not altogether different. It is a little less water-like and a little more air-like. Move over a bit farther. Again, you are in an area that is a little less water-like and a little more air-like. You are used to the water-like properties and can see how the air-like properties are similar to them. Now, you can find some strategies to cope as you travel farther into the more air-like areas.

Find ways to see your pre- and post- mastectomy body in terms of their similarities. A new chest area can be considered as just somewhat more flat, hard, numb, or perky than it was previously. These are not necessarily good changes, but the mind knows how to handle changes in degree. It does not know what to do with a totally unknown scenario. This is why we are so afraid of the unknown.

## 3. Keep A Good Thought.

Consider a very simple, but very useful way of looking at how you can help yourself heal. Good thoughts create good chemicals. Bad thoughts create bad chemicals. Your thoughts do have power. They create your reality in a concrete, chemical way. This is why having a good attitude is a real advantage.

## 4. Make Connections.

We are social animals. We need to see how things connect and relate to each other. More importantly, we need to feel connected to our world. We need relationships with those around us. When we are in harmony with ourselves, others and the world, we are at our best.

Find balance and harmony from the inside out through:

Meditation
Prayer
Keeping a Journal
Yoga
T'ai Chi
Exercise
Humor
Getting professional counseling.

Find balance and harmony from the outside in through:

Enjoying friends – strengthen relationships
Communing with nature – spend time outside
Volunteering – reach out to others
Forgiving – feel expansive
Showing appreciation – feel humble
Touching – feel connected to others
Smelling – concentrate on how a scent brings together
    many memories
Hearing – experience harmony through music
Seeing – see that the whole is greater than the sum of the
    parts through art
Eating plenty of ice cream – taste the sweetness of life.

# AFTERWORD

"*In spite of illness, in spite even of the archenemy sorrow, one **can** remain alive long past the usual date of disintegration if one is unafraid of change, insatiable in intellectual curiosity, interested in big things, and happy in small ways.*"
—Edith Wharton